Quick and Easy Recipes

34 Healthy & Tasty Meals for Busy Moms to Feed the Whole Family!

by Olivia Rogers

Copyright © 2017 By Olivia Rogers
All rights reserved. No part of this book may be reproduced in any form without permission in writing from the author. No part of this publication may be reproduced or transmitted in any form or by any means, mechanic, electronic, photocopying, recording, by any storage or retrieval system, or transmitted by email without the permission in writing from the author and publisher.
For information regarding permissions write to author at Olivia@TheMenuAtHome.com
Reviewers may quote brief passages in review.

Please note that credit for the images used in this book go to the respective owners. You can view this at:
TheMenuAtHome.com/image-list

Olivia Rogers
TheMenuAtHome.com

Table of Contents

Introduction _____ 5
1. Creamy Black Bean Chicken Soup _____ 6
2. Best Baked Beans _____ 8
3. Grilled Cheese _____ 10
4. Cashew Chicken Crockpot Dish _____ 12
5. Yum Egg Boats _____ 15
6. Lemony Cream Cheese Pancake with Blueberries ___ 18
7. Cheesy Chicken Bagel Pizza _____ 21
8. Best Baked Mozzarella Bites _____ 23
9. Linguine with Easy Meat Sauce _____ 25
10. Creamy Ranch Style Dip _____ 27
11. Tomato Basil Soup _____ 29
12. Popcorn Balls _____ 31
13. Beef and Broccoli Bowls _____ 33
14. Crisp Stuffed Apples _____ 35
15. Maple Roast Vegetables _____ 37
16. Po-Taco _____ 39
17. Corn Muffins _____ 41
18. Panko Crusted Fish Sticks _____ 43
19. Mushroom Quesadillas _____ 46
20. Crispy Onion Rings _____ 48
21. Sushi Sandwiches _____ 50
22. Tomato Pico De Gallo _____ 52
23. Summer Corn and Tomato Salad _____ 54

24. Sweet Potato Pancake Stack _____ 56

25. Zucchini Mini Muffins _____ 58

26. Sunflower Granola Breakfast Parfaits _____ 61

27. Swedish Meatballs _____ 64

28. Apple and Bacon Pita Pizzas _____ 66

29. Peach and Blueberry Oatmeal _____ 68

30. Baked Apples _____ 70

31. Pumpkin Risotto _____ 72

32. Raspberry Ricotta Cake _____ 74

33. Cashew Chicken _____ 76

34. Peanut Butter Hummus Along with Cucumber Dips _____ 79

Final Words _____ 81

Disclaimer _____ 83

Introduction

Everyone loves a tasty meal and moms in particular may have a hard time trying to come up with great recipes to keep kids happy.

If you are looking for some really tasty and healthy recipes that can be cooked in little or no time, this is the ultimate book to have.

We are going to offer some of the best recipes that will allow you to make your family proud of your culinary skills.

So, let us get going and learn how to cook some of the finest meals which the whole family will love to devour.

1. Creamy Black Bean Chicken Soup

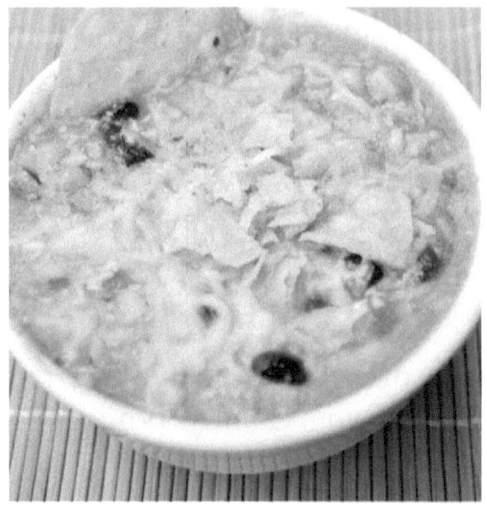

There's no better starter than a perfectly cooked soup. Chicken soups are always a favorite among people because it is loaded with proteins and tastes absolutely delicious as well.

Ingredients

- 1 cup chicken broth
- 1 can of drained corn
- 2 chicken breasts
- 1 can of black beans which has been drained and rinsed thoroughly
- 1 package of taco seasoning

- 1 cup salsa

- Tortilla chips

- ½ cup each of cheddar cheese and sour cream (both these items are optional)

Method

1. Take a crock pot and place chicken in it. Now add the broth along with corn salsa, beans and even taco seasoning over the chicken. Cook the whole mixture on high for 3 hours.

2. Now remove the chicken and shred it. You can re-add chicken later. Feel free to add sour cream and cheese as per your needs to the Crockpot. Make sure to stir it until the whole paste is smooth. Serve the soup along with tortilla chips for extra taste.

Tips

If you are a little skeptical of weight gain and calorie content, you should skip sour cream and cheddar cheese as a cup of soup with cheese and sour cream contains as much as 568 calories. However, your body does get the essential 43.5 gm protein in the single cup serving too which is great for growing children.

2. Best Baked Beans

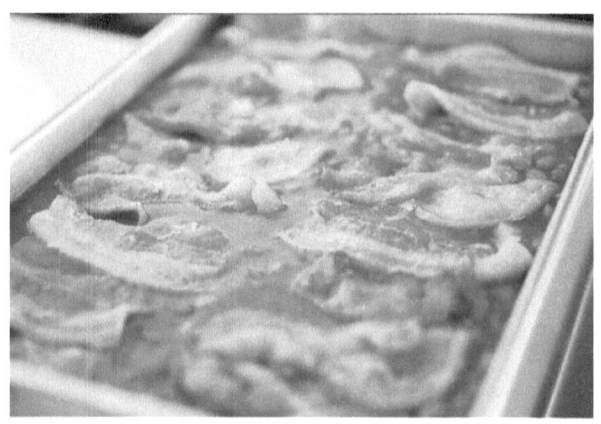

Those who love bacon and beef (as we all do) will never cease to love this dish. It is a heavy meal, but worth every bit of time and effort you put into making it.

Ingredients

- 1 pound of ground beef which is thoroughly cooked; drained and even crumbled

- 1 pound of well cooked bacon

- 2 tablespoons of bacon drippings

- 14-ounce cans of kidney beans, white beans and even pork and beans each

- 3 small onions

- 1 cup ketchup

- 1 cup sugar (light brown)

- 3 tablespoons of yellow mustard

- ½ cup of molasses

Method

1. Take all the beans and drain them, taking care to leave just one can of pork and beans.

2. Now pour all the ingredients in a Crockpot and heat it. Heat the dish for nearly 4 hours on high and you are all set to enjoy the dish.

Tips

Make sure to use a big Crockpot as the ingredients listed are quite a lot. So, having a small Crockpot could turn out to be a little tedious. You can leave the dish on high and attend other work as well. This recipe offers 16 servings.

3. Grilled Cheese

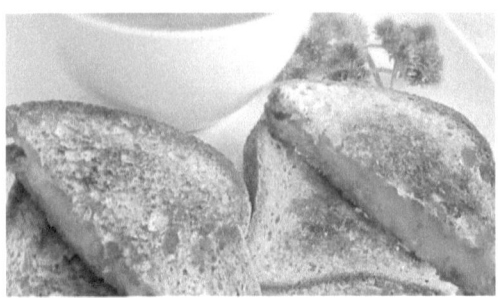

Nothing quite beats the morning hunger as efficiently as a well prepared grilled cheese toast.

Ingredients

- 2 slices of white bread
- Little butter
- Mayonnaise
- A couple of slices of American cheese
- Pepper

Method

1. Take 2 slices of white bread and put them on a cutting board. Evenly spread mayonnaise on top of it. Take a small nonstick skillet and heat it over medium flame. Pour a little butter on it and wait for the butter to melt.

2. Now, place one slice of bread and make sure the side smeared with mayonnaise is placed downwards. Add a few slices of American cheese and season it with pepper. Add the second slice of bread keeping the mayonnaise side up.

3. When the underside turns somewhat golden brown in color, turn over the sandwich and add butter to the skillet. Press the sandwich closely to allow the cheese to melt. When the second side attains a golden-brown color too, the sandwich has been prepared.

Tips

The dish is best served along with tomato soup as sandwiches really blend well along with a soup. You can also use cheddar instead of American cheese based upon your preferences.

4. Cashew Chicken Crockpot Dish

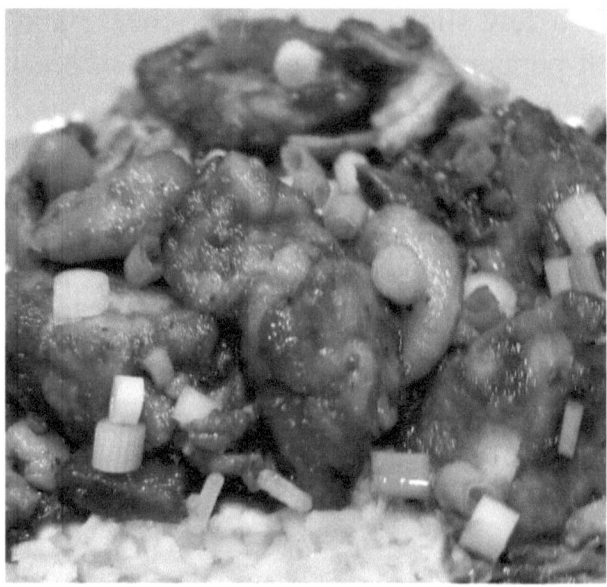

If you love Chinese takeout but don't want to harm your health, this is an excellent prepare at home dish which you can use as a substitute.

Ingredients

- 2 chicken breasts that have been cut into smaller pieces

- 1 to 2 cups of frozen broccoli that have been cut into tiny even pieces

- ½ cup of unsalted cashews

- 1 cup of sliced carrot

- 1 tablespoon olive oil
- 3 tablespoon ketchup
- ½ cup soy sauce
- 4 tablespoon of rice wine vinegar
- 1 tablespoon of brown sugar
- 1 tablespoon of ginger paste
- ½ cup water or even chicken broth
- 1 minced garlic clove
- ¼ teaspoon red pepper
- Salt and pepper, as per taste

Method

1. Take the Crockpot and layer chicken, cashews and vegetables in it. Combine all other ingredients except water and then pour the same over chicken in your Crockpot.

2. Feel free to add water or broth to the mixture to ensure that it is completely covered. Keep it on high and let it cook for 2 to 4 hours.

Tips

It would be a great idea to roast the cashews before adding them as it makes them crisp and therefore tastier. Also, it is completely alright to use fresh broccoli rather than frozen ones.

5. Yum Egg Boats

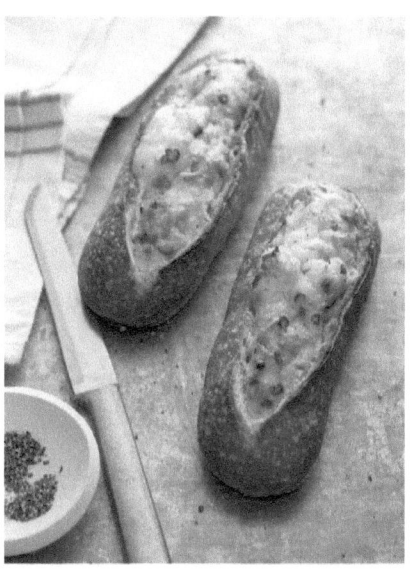

If you are really crammed for time and you still want to cook something healthy and delicious, the egg boat definitely wins the argument.

Ingredients

- 4 demi sourdough baguettes

- 8 eggs

- 3 thinly sliced green onions

- 1 complete package of spicy pork sausage links (7 ounce)

- 8 ounces of grated pepper jack cheese

- ½ cup of heavy cream

- Salt and pepper

Method

1. Preheat your oven to 350 F. Take the sourdough baguettes and cut them by pulling out the middle. You should leave ½ inch of bread on the sides and the bottom as well. As per the directions offered in the package, prepare the sausage.

2. Now, cut down the links into tiny pieces and keep them aside. Take a medium sized bowl and beat eggs and cream together. Pour in the remaining ingredients along with the sausage. Make it a point to divide the mixture and put it evenly in the baguette boat.

3. Keep all 4 baguettes on a baking sheet and allow them to bake for nearly 25 to 30 minutes. Let the boats cool down for 10 minutes and then you can cut them and serve.

Tips

Eggs are a great choice for children as it helps in their growth. It is rich in protein and gives the body the much-needed strength. Owing to the presence of cheese, children are much more likely to enjoy this meal as it is definitely tasty.

Read This FIRST - 100% FREE BONUS

FOR A LIMITED TIME ONLY – Get Olivia's best-selling book *"The #1 Cookbook: Over 170+ of the Most Popular Recipes Across 7 Different Cuisines!"* absolutely FREE!

Readers have absolutely loved this book because of the wide variety of recipes. It is highly recommended you check these recipes out and see what you can add to your home menu!

Once again, as a big thank-you for downloading this book, I'd like to offer it to you *100% FREE for a LIMITED TIME ONLY!*

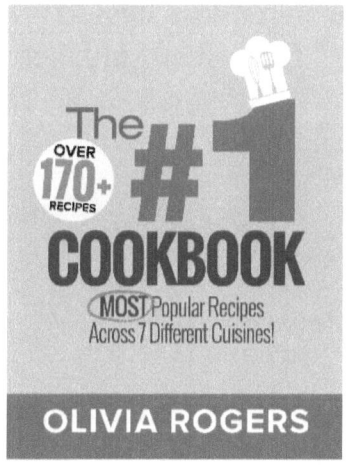

Get your free copy at:

TheMenuAtHome.com/Bonus

6. Lemony Cream Cheese Pancake with Blueberries

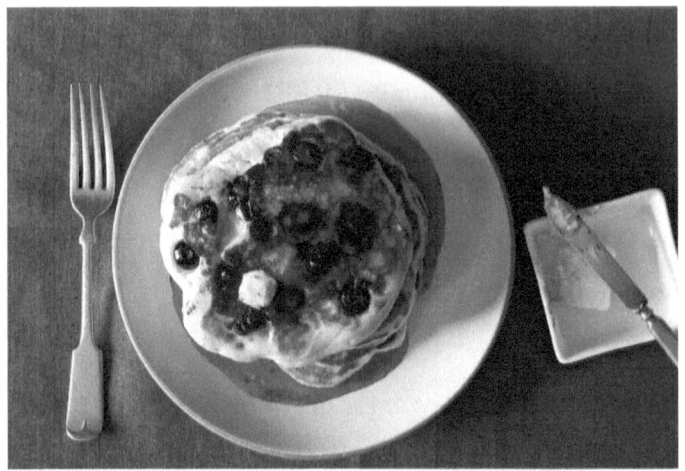

This is one of the yummiest desserts which your family will love to devour. The taste of blueberries in pancake is a complete bliss and it is a must have recipe for all those who have a sweet tooth.

Ingredients

- 1 ½ cup of flour
- 1 tablespoon of sugar and baking powder each
- 2 large eggs
- 6 ounces of cut up cream cheese
- ½ teaspoon baking soda

- 3 teaspoons melted butter

- 1 cup buttermilk

- 1 large lemon

- 1 ½ cups of blueberries. They can be either fresh or frozen.

- 2 tablespoon lemon juice

- 1 pinch salt

- 1 teaspoon vanilla

Method

1. Take a medium bowl and mix flour, baking soda, sugar baking powder and salt in it. Take another bowl and mix egg yolk along with buttermilk.

2. Now add cream cheese to it and mix it thoroughly until you find small lumps of cheese curds. Mix melted butter, lemon juice and vanilla to it. Add the dry ingredients to the wet mixture and then stir them thoroughly to combine.

3. Mix the two egg whites until it becomes stiff and fold it gently in a batter. Take a pan and put it over medium high heat. Lower the heat a little and then add butter to the pan.

4. Add berries to the spread butter. Cover it with batter. If the mixture begins to sizzle, lower down the heat. Let them puff and then you can turn them and leave for a couple of minutes. Serve along with maple syrup or jam.

Tips

The cooking time might be a little higher. If you are not skeptical of the extra calories, you can also use chocolate syrup along with the pancake.

7. Cheesy Chicken Bagel Pizza

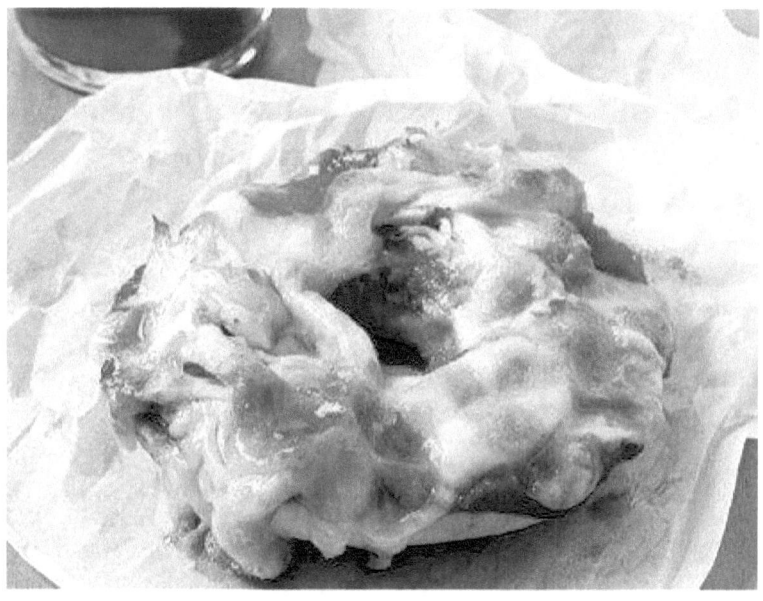

Pizza is the eternal favorite among children and if you can add cheesy chicken to the mix, the dish can't get any better.

Ingredients

- 4 ½ inch and 2 ¼ ounce plain bagels; 2 in number which have been sliced into halves.

- ½ cup marinara sauce with low sodium composition

- 1 cup pre-shredded mozzarella cheese which is part skimmed

- 1 cup shredded chicken breast

Method

1. Take the boiler and preheat it. Place the bagel halves on a baking sheet and cut them with the sides facing up. Boil it for 2 minutes until it is lightly toasted. Apply 2 tablespoons of marinara sauce on the bagel halves that have been cut.

2. On each half, add $1/4^{th}$ cup of chicken and sprinkle nearly 14 cups of cheese. Boil the bagel halves for a couple of minutes until the cheese begins to melt.

Tips

It is the marinara sauce that truly does the trick in the recipe as it gives a very characteristic flavor to the whole pizza.

8. Best Baked Mozzarella Bites

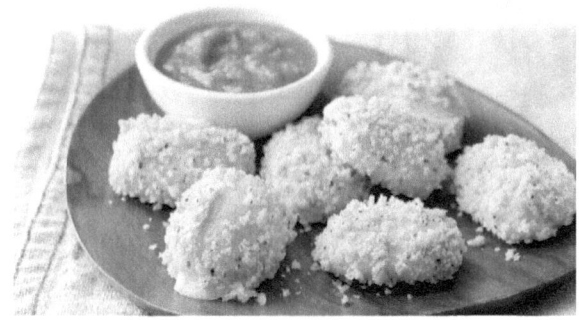

This makes an excellent quick snack for children. Cooking this will ensure that your kids will have something to look forward to when they come back from school.

Ingredients

- 1/3 cup of Japanese breadcrumbs

- 1 ounce sticks that are part skimmed in mozzarella string cheese; 3 in number

- ¼ cup marinara sauce with low sodium

- 3 tablespoon egg substitutes

- Cooking spray

Method

1. Preheat the oven to 425 degrees. Take a midsized skillet and put it to medium heat. Add 1/3rd cup of Japanese breadcrumbs to the pan and cook it for 2

minutes. Make sure to stir it frequently. Remove the heating source and place the breadcrumb in a shallow dish.

2. Take mozzarella sticks and cut them into pieces measuring 1 inch each. Take every single piece and dip it in egg substitute and dredge the same in breadcrumbs.

3. Place the cheese on the baking sheet and coat it with a layer of cooking spray. Bake at 425 degrees for 3 minutes. Take a bowl and pour marinara sauce in it. Keep it in microwave at high for 1 minute. Serve it with the mozzarella pieces.

Tips

When you are cutting the mozzarella sticks, you have to be sure that they are evenly diced. If the mozzarella sticks are uneven; it will spoil the overall look of the dish.

9. Linguine with Easy Meat Sauce

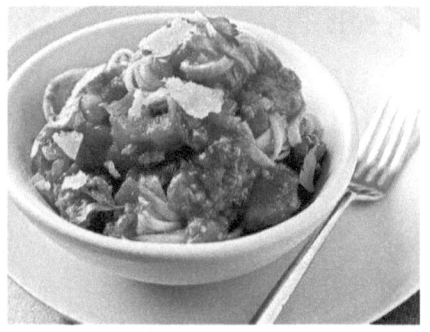

This dish has been designed with a difference and if you are looking to cook something special and unique, you can't go wrong with this recipe.

Ingredients

- A 9-ounce package of fresh linguine
- 1/2-pound ground beef, extra lean
- 1 tablespoon of fresh garlic which has been nicely minced
- 1 can of drained diced tomatoes weighing 14.5 ounces.
- ½ cup pre-chopped onion
- 1 teaspoon dried oregano
- 3 tablespoons tomato paste

- 1 ounce of shaved parmigiano- reggiano cheese

- ¼ teaspoon salt

- 1 tablespoon of fresh parsley leaves which are flat leaf

Method

1. Follow the directions in the package and cook your pasta as usual. Take a large skillet and put it over medium to high heat. Add onion, oregano, garlic, beef and salt to the skillet and cook it for 5 minutes until you find that the beef has gained a brownish color.

2. Pour in the tomato paste and stir the whole thing. Cook it for 1 minute. Make sure to frequently stir the whole mixture. Add tomatoes to the mixture and bring it to boil. Keep cooking for a minute.

3. Now, reduce the heat to medium low and cook for 3 minutes. Do so until you find the mixture thicken. Pour it over pasta and serve along with parsley and a little cheese topping.

Tips

When you are making this dish, you can choose to have your own style of pasta. Be particular with the seasoning you include in the recipe or else the sauce will fail to give the apt flavor.

10. Creamy Ranch Style Dip

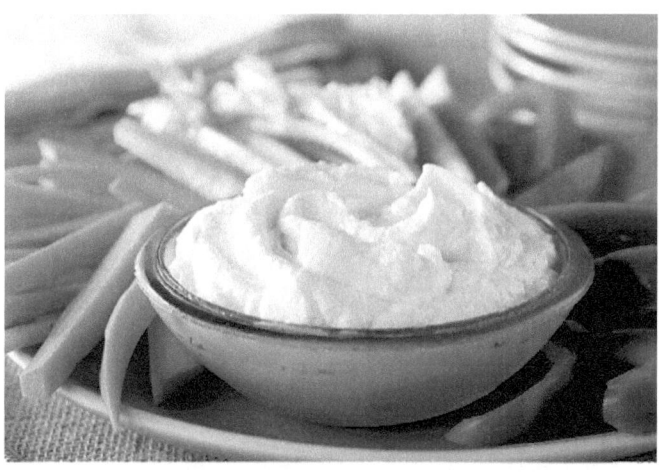

If you love to spice up your food with the right kind of recipe, this one here is going to give you the best taste you could ask for.

Ingredients

- 4 ounces of softened cream cheese
- 2 tablespoons of chopped fresh parsley
- 3 tablespoons of nonfat buttermilk
- 1 teaspoon of chopped fresh dill
- ¼ teaspoon of onion powder, black pepper and salt.
- ½ teaspoon of fresh garlic

Method

1. Take a small bowl and mix cream, cheese and buttermilk in it.

2. Stir it with a whisk until it is perfectly blended. Pour in the remaining ingredients and stir it thoroughly.

Tips

This recipe takes into account most of the low-fat ingredients which means that despite the presence of cheese, it will not be very high in calorie and is therefore a healthy choice.

11. Tomato Basil Soup

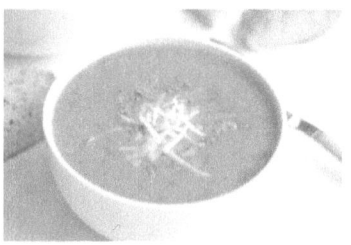

There are a few appetizers as great as tomato basil soup. It is ideal before a big lunch and can be cooked easily too.

Ingredients

- 1 ½ cups of onion that are pre-chopped
- ¾ cup of fresh basil, finely chopped
- 1 tablespoon of extra virgin olive oil
- 3 chopped garlic cloves
- 2 cups of 1% low fat milk
- 1 halved garlic clove
- ¼ teaspoon of salt
- ¼ teaspoon black pepper
- 1 can of un-drained diced tomatoes weighing 28 ounces

- ½ cup of less fat cream cheese; 4 ounces

- 12 slices of French bread

- 1 ounce of shredded Asiago cheese

Method

1. Preheat the boiler keeping it to high. Pour olive oil in a sauce and heat it at medium. Add onion and sauté it for three minutes. Pour garlic and cook it for a minute.

2. Add basil and tomatoes and oil the mixture. Stir the cheese in the mix until it melts. Pour the whole mixture in a blender and keep blending until the paste is smooth.

3. Pour back the mixture in the pan and stir it with milk, salt and pepper. Cook on medium high flame for a couple of minutes. Put the breads on a baking sheet and apply a little spray as coating. Broil it for a minute. Rub a little garlic on the toasted side and then turn the bread over. Top it with Asiago and broil for another minute.

Tips

Basil is an excellent ingredient and has an extremely high nutritional value. Using basil can improve your overall health as it strengthens your immunity.

12. Popcorn Balls

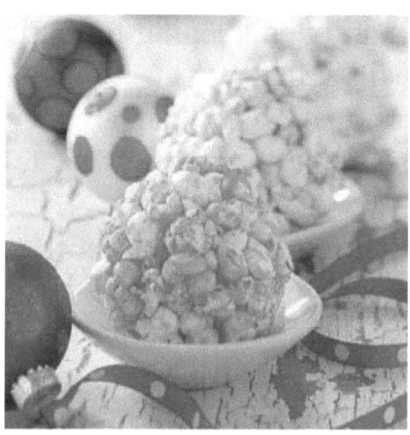

If you want to cook a quick meal which your kids will love to eat, this recipe fits the equation. It is so much fun giving little popcorns a big twist.

Ingredients

- 1 tablespoon of canola oil
- 2 tablespoons of unsalted butter
- 3 tablespoons of unpopped popcorn kernels
- 1 cup oat cereal which is honey nut toasted
- ¼ cup salted peanuts that have been dry roasted
- 2 ¼ cup mini marshmallows
- 1 ounce of pretzel sticks

Method

1. Heat oil in an oven keeping it on medium heat. Add kernels to it and cover it. Cook it for 4 minutes. Make sure to shake the pan frequently. Take butter in the pan and melt it over low heat.

2. Add marshmallows to it and let it cook for a couple minutes. Remove the heating after it. Add 3 cups of popcorn and other remaining ingredients as well. Stir it thoroughly. Let it cool for 2 minutes and you can make 3-inch balls from it.

Tips

Popcorns always make excellent snacks as they do not make your stomach heavy. They are light and can be easily digested.

13. Beef and Broccoli Bowls

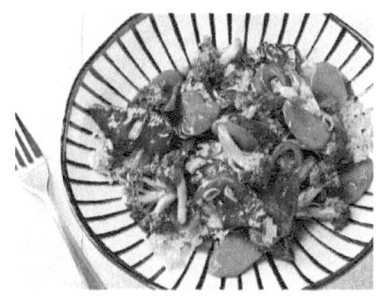

The combination of beef and broccoli is mesmerizing, and this recipe is sure to leave you happy that you made the right cooking choice. Broccoli is an excellent health food.

Ingredients

- 1 bag of long grain rice weighing 3 ½ ounces
- 1 boneless sirloin streak which has been cut into thin strips
- ¼ cup soy sauce which is low in sodium
- 2 teaspoons canola oil
- 2 teaspoons dark sesame oil
- 1 cup of chopped carrot
- 2 cups broccoli florets
- 1 tablespoon of cornstarch

- 1 cup red onion which is vertically sliced

- ½ cup water

- 1/3 cup green onions which have been sliced

Method

1. Use the package directions and cook rice accordingly. Take a medium bowl and mix cornstarch, soy sauce and hoisin in it. Add beef and toss it to make thick coat. Remove the beef and reserve the marinade.

2. Now add the beef to the pan and cook it for 2 minutes until it gets a little brown color. Now remove the beef from the pan and add broccoli and pour sesame oil to add more ingredients. Cook for 4 minutes until the broccoli becomes crisp.

3. Add a little marinade to the pan and then boil it. Cook it for a minute. Add beef to the pan and cook it for another minute. Sprinkle green onions and serve it with rice.

Tips

The heating time is very important in this dish. Make sure that you let the ingredients cook thoroughly so that you can get the most out of the taste.

14. Crisp Stuffed Apples

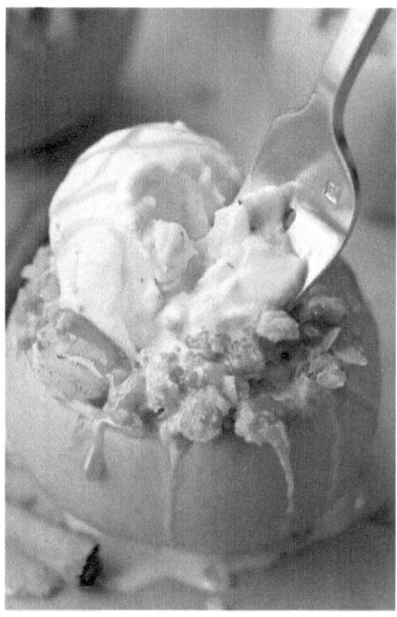

We are all aware of how eating apples are considered to be one of the healthiest habits you could have. This recipe is good at helping people enjoy apple with its nutritional intake and an added taste.

Ingredients

- 4 to 6 pieces of apple
- 1 cup of brown sugar
- ¾ cup of chopped pecans
- 1 cup margarine

- ½ teaspoon cinnamon

- 1 cup of instant oats

Method

1. Take a medium sized bowl and mix the different apple crisp ingredients in it. Wash your apples and stuff them with the apple crisp mixture. Spray the cook pot with a nonstick spray and then place the apples in it.

2. Sprinkle the rest of the topping over the apples and let the remaining leftover fall down to the bottom of your pot. Cover the whole thing and cook it on low for 6 to 8 hours. Cut them into half and you can top it with your favorite ice cream flavor, if needed.

Tips

If you choose to have this dish along with the ice cream, it can be a little calorie rich. However, if you are more bothered about the taste, this is definitely the best way to approach.

15. Maple Roast Vegetables

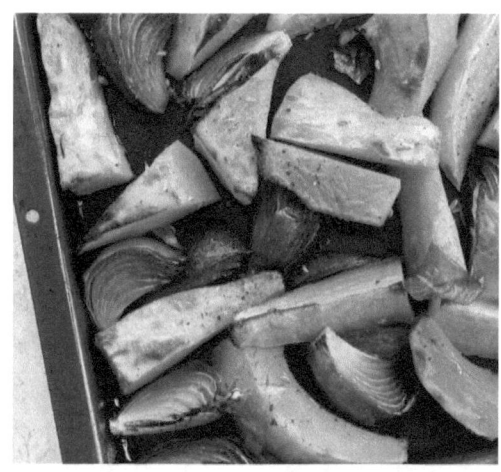

It is no surprise that vegetables are the healthiest food people can have. When you are looking to make a quick breakfast, which has a very high nutritional value, this is the recipe you need to use.

Ingredients

- 7 peeled carrots that have been sliced into half through the length and cut into 2-inch sized pieces

- 1 yellow onion that has been cut into wedges

- 2 red bell peppers that have been cut into large chunks

- 1 unpeeled delicate squash which has been cut lengthwise and has the seeds removed. Cut them into shapes resembling half-moons.

- 2 teaspoon oil

- 1 tablespoon sea salt

- 2 tablespoon maple syrup

Method

1. Preheat oven to 245 degrees. Take a bowl and add all the ingredients to it. Toss it such that you can coat all the vegetables.

2. Put the vegetables on a tray that is lined by a foil sheet and roast it for nearly 50 minutes. Make sure to store the mixture halfway through and keep doing so until the ingredients turn golden. The dish is now ready to be served.

Tips

You can always do a little garnishing at the end to make the dish good to look at. This is a healthy dish as it is packed with important nutrient rich vegetables like carrot which is extremely rich in vitamin A

16. Po-Taco

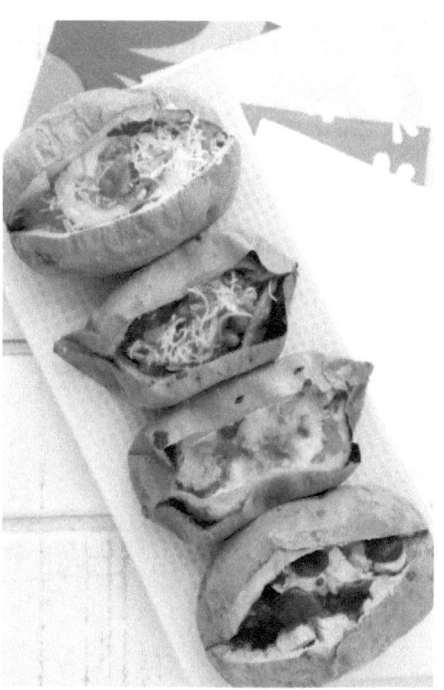

Just as the name implies, this dish is going to let you have a blend of potato and tacos in a brilliant mix. Those who can't even comprehend of what these two items together will look like; you should definitely give this a try.

Ingredients

- 4 sweet potatoes

- In order to make the filling for the potato, you can use either of the following options.

- Chicken chili along with cheddar cheese

- Chicken along with bbq sauce

- Pesto, Greek yogurt and manchego cheese

- Refried beans along with sour cream and salsa

Method

1. Preheat the oven to 400 degrees Fahrenheit. Make numerous holes in the sides of the potatoes and then place it on a baking sheet which has been lined with foil. Bake it for an hour.

2. Slice the potatoes through the middle and extract half of the inner flesh. Fill it with the options you want and take a bite.

Tips

This isn't the most calorie friendly dish but once in a while, when you are looking to have the most delicious meal, this is certainly the best choice you have.

17. Corn Muffins

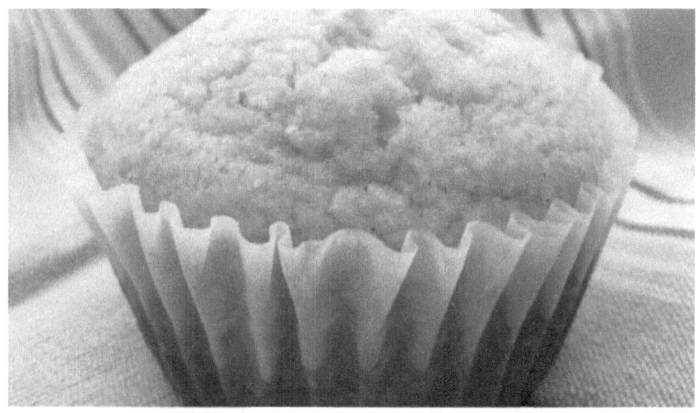

If you are really short of time and you want to make a quick meal, this is the perfect recipe. Those who love corn will absolutely crave for this dish.

Ingredients

- 1 ¾ cup cornmeal
- 2 large eggs
- ¾ cup of flour
- ¼ cup vegetable oil
- 1 teaspoon baking soda
- ½ teaspoon salt
- 1 tablespoon baking powder

- ¼ cup honey or agrave

- 1 ½ cup buttermilk

- 24 greased mini muffin cups

Method

1. Preheat the oven to 425 degrees. Take all the dry ingredients and mix them thoroughly in a bowl. Take a separate bowl and thoroughly mix all other wet ingredients in it.

2. Add the cornmeal mixture to the wet ingredients and combine it thoroughly. Take 24 greased mini muffin cups and pour the mixture to it. Bake it for 15 minutes. Let it cool for some time and serve.

Tips

Muffins offer a lot of scope and it allows you to be creative. There are a lot of different fillings you can come up with. Corn muffins are very soft and dissolve on the mouth very quickly.

18. Panko Crusted Fish Sticks

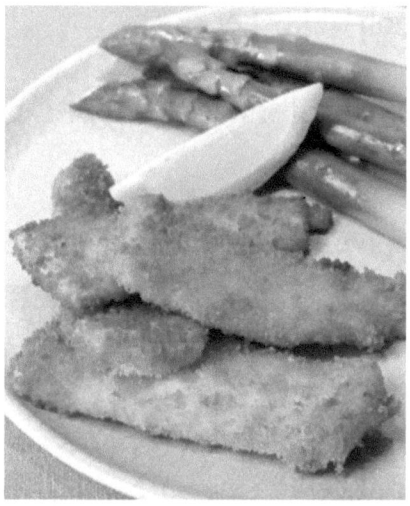

If you are looking for a good dinner recipe which your family will love to gorge upon, you can try this recipe out.

Ingredients

- 1 tablespoon of 2% reduced fat milk

- 2 lightly beaten large eggs

- 1 cup panko

- 1 pound of halibut fillets which have been cut into 20 strips measuring 1 inches each.

- 3/8 teaspoon of freshly grounded black pepper

- ¼ cup light sour cream

- 2 teaspoons minced capers

- 3/8 teaspoon of kosher salt

- 2 tablespoons of finely chopped bread and butter pickles

- 3 tablespoon canola mayonnaise

- 2 tablespoons divided canola oil

Method

1. Take a large bowl and combine both milk and eggs in it. Stir it thoroughly. Add fish to the mixture and toss it such that the mixture gets coated. Take a large zip top bag and add Panko, ¼ teaspoon of salt and same amount of pepper in it. Add fish to the panko mixture and then seal the bag. Shake the bag gently such that fish is coated.

2. Take a large nonstick skillet and put it over medium to high heat. Add 1 tablespoon oil to the pan and swirl it for coating. Add half of the fish and cook for 4 minutes until the fish turns brownish at all sides. Repeat the same process with 1 tablespoon oil and the rest of the fish.

3. Take a small bowl and mix sour cream along with capers, mayonnaise, pickles and the remaining 1/8 teaspoon of salt. Serve the sauce along with the fish.

Tips

Mayonnaise plays a very important role in making the sauce because it will give you the right flavor. Also, make it a point to cook the fish thoroughly because semi-cooked fish will not serve your need.

19. Mushroom Quesadillas

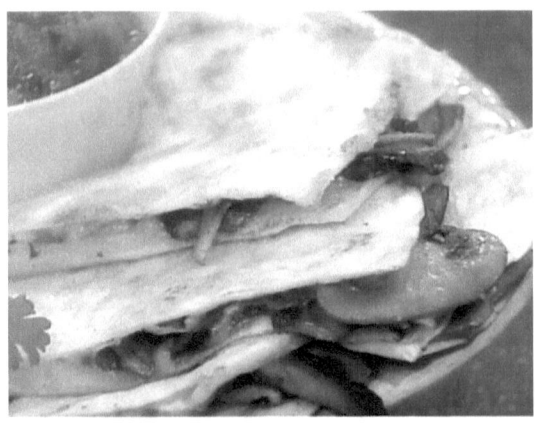

If you have guests coming at home and you need to impress them with a quick recipe, this is the perfect choice. Quesadillas when coked right make an excellent meal which leaves people asking for more.

Ingredients

- 2 tortillas

- ½ cup sliced mushrooms

- ½ cup of grated cheese

Method

1. Take a skillet and put it over medium heat. Take the tortillas and put it in tea pan and let it cook for a minute. Flip over the tortillas and sprinkle cheese over it.

2. When the cheese begins to melt, pour mushroom over half of the total and then fold them into halves. Cook both the sides for a couple of minutes each. Now, remove the quesadillas and add the stuffing based on your choice.

Tips

It is important to pick the best choice of stuffing because the taste of quesadillas comes out best when you team them with the perfect stuffing. Also, make sure that the cheese melts through because clusters of cheese in between will take away the charm of the dish.

20. Crispy Onion Rings

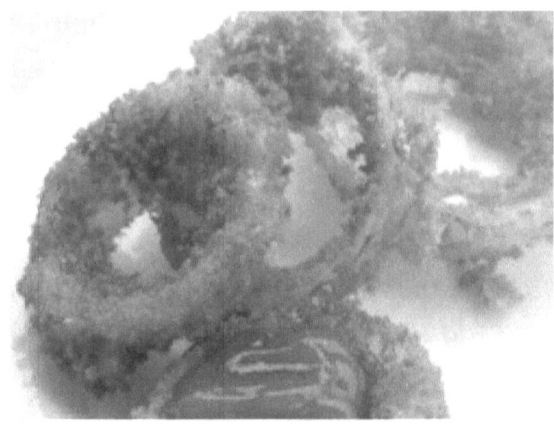

This dish can be cooked in as less as 30 minutes and it is ideal for serving 4 people. You will enjoy the taste of the dish as the method of preparation gives the right zing to it.

Ingredients

- 1 large sweet Maui onion
- 2 teaspoons of divided salt
- 1 ½ cup of plain breadcrumbs
- ¾ cup buttermilk
- Canola oil spray

Method

1. Preheat the oven to 425 degrees. Take onions and cut them into round shape measuring ½ inches and

separate them into rings. Take a bowl and mix buttermilk with 1 teaspoon of salt.

2. Take another bowl and place breadcrumbs in it. To this, add another teaspoon of salt. Place the onion rings in the buttermilk mixture and then pour it in the breadcrumb mixture such that it covers both sides of the onion thoroughly.

3. Now place the onion rings over a baking sheet. Pour cooking oil spray over it in small quantity. Bake the dish for 20 to 25 minutes and make sure to turn them thoroughly in between. Bake it until you get a light brown color. Serve it.

Tips

Make it a point to dice the onion evenly. It can take a little effort and practice to make exact onion rings, but it is important to do so because it is the perfectly carved rings which make the dish special.

21. Sushi Sandwiches

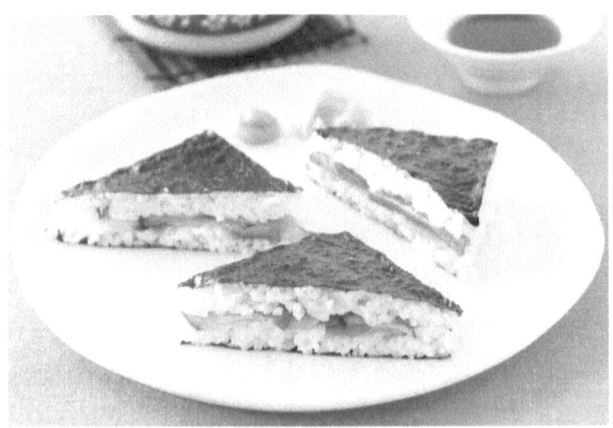

This is perhaps the quickest meal which you can make. It takes less than 5 minutes to cook it and serves a great way to satiate your appetite.

Ingredients

- 3-piece sandwich bread (whole wheat)

- 1 grated carrot

- 1 can of tuna

- 1 cucumber that has been cut into long sticks

- 1 tablespoon mayonnaise

- 1 teaspoon chopped capers

- ½ teaspoon Dijon mustard

Method

1. Take a slice of bread and cut the crusts. Take a rolling pin and roll out the slice as thin as possible. Take a bowl and add tuna, mayonnaise, Dijon and capers to it. Stir the ingredients such that it combines efficiently. Spread an extremely thin layer of mayonnaise on every single slice of bread. Take 1/3 of the tuna mixture and spread it onto the half of the bread.

2. Now, take some cucumber sticks and grated carrot and pour it over the tuna mixture. However, do not overstuff the roll. Tightly roll the mixture to one side of the bread and then press it and seal it up making a roll. Cut the roll into 4 pieces and repeat the same with your bread and tuna mixture.

Tips

This is an excellent dish because carrots are an extremely rich source of vitamin A. By choosing to add carrot to this sandwich; you will be able to make a nutritious breakfast.

22. Tomato Pico De Gallo

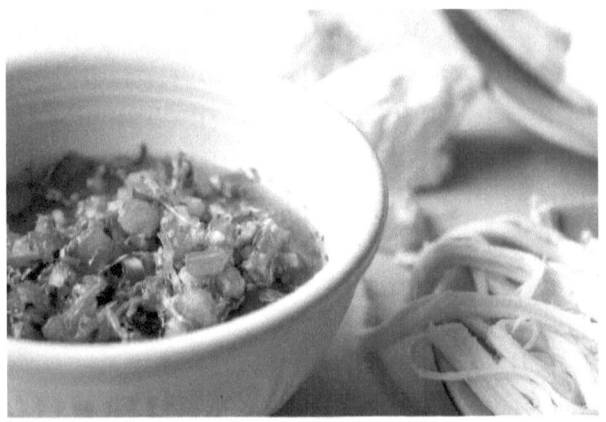

If you are looking for a tangy recipe that can satiate your taste buds, this is definitely a good choice. Those who have fetish for tomatoes are going to love what this dish has to offer.

Ingredients

- 1 small red onion

- 2 cups of heirloom tomatoes which are seeded and chopped

- ¼ cup of chopped cilantro

- Juice made from 2 limes

- 1 chili pepper with removed and minced seeds

- ½ teaspoon kosher salt

Method

1. Take a bowl and combine all ingredients. Let it sit for 30 minutes such that the different flavors can combine.

2. Serve it as a dip along with tortilla chips or you can also pour it on along with a grilled chicken or a fish.

Tips

This recipe is best used as an add-on for different dishes. It can really add the extra zing and flavor and make you crave for the meals. It is best suited with tortillas

23. Summer Corn and Tomato Salad

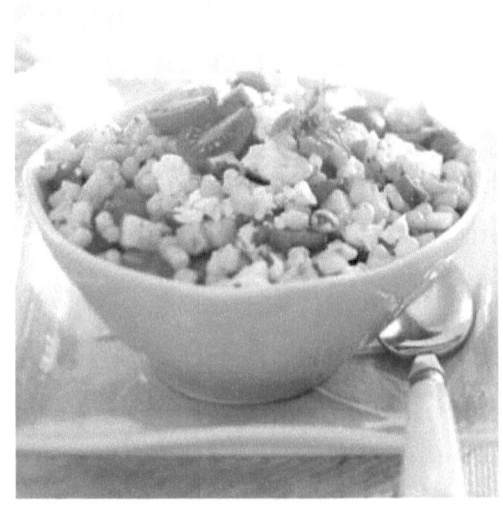

Salads make an excellent breakfast and they are very rich in nutritional value as well. The best thing about salads is that they can be prepared in little or no time.

Ingredients

- 20 corn ears
- 6 fresh ripe tomatoes
- Oil
- Salt
- Pepper
- paprika

Method

1. Take a charcoal grill and put it to high heat. Take a large pot and add salt and water to it. Make sure to boil the mixture thoroughly. Take the corns and cut all their ears into half. This makes it easy to remove the kernels. Make it a point to blanch the corn until they turn bright yellow. Remove it from the pot and then let it dry for few minutes.

2. Now, head to the grill and place all corn on it. Try and burn each side a little so that you can have a mix of burned and unburned kernels. Take a large bowl and add diced tomatoes to it.

3. Remove the corns from the grill and make it a point to cut down all the kernels. Add the corn to the bowl and pour pepper, salt and a tablespoon of paprika. Now, add olive oil to it and mix it until it's lightly coated. Adjust the seasoning as per need and serve it.

Tips

There is a lot of taste in the seasoning and you should make it a point to add it in an accurate manner. Eating salads is one of the best ways to stay healthy and you can team it with your lunch as well.

24. Sweet Potato Pancake Stack

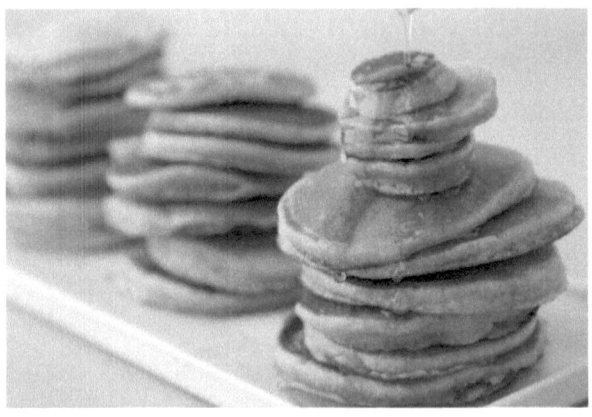

There are very few people who don't like pancakes and when you blend it with sweet potato, the result is stupefying.

Ingredients

- 1 cup white whole wheat flour

- 1 large egg

- 2 teaspoons baking powder

- 1 ¼ cups milk

- 1 cup sweet potato puree

- ½ teaspoon ground cinnamon

- 1 tablespoon vegetable oil

- ¼ teaspoon ground nutmeg

- 1 tablespoon brown sugar

- ½ teaspoon salt

Method

1. Take a bowl and mix flour, cinnamon, salt, nutmeg, baking powder. Take another bowl and mix all other remaining ingredients. Now slowly add dry ingredients to the mix of wet ingredients and keep on mixing them until they combine thoroughly.

2. Take a large skillet and put it to medium heat. Now, lightly coat it with oil. Pour nearly 1 tablespoon of pancake mixture on the skillet and out as many pancakes as possible in the skillet. Cook for a couple of minutes. Flip over the pancakes and then cook for another minute.

Tips

When you are preparing this dish, you have to be very careful when you are mixing the wet and the dry ingredients because rushing through it can lead to a lot of troubles.

25. Zucchini Mini Muffins

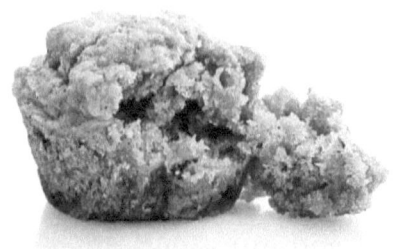

You can cook it for either breakfast or snacks. They make an excellent quick recipe and are always fun to eat. Not everyone loves zucchini but if they do, this is going to be one tempting thing to watch out for.

Ingredients

- 6 ounces of all-purpose flour measuring about 1 1/3 cups
- 1 teaspoon baking powder
- ½ teaspoon salt
- ½ cup packed dark brown sugar
- 2/3 cup shredded zucchini
- 1 teaspoon ground cinnamon
- 1 teaspoon vanilla extract

- 2 tablespoon melted butter

- ¼ teaspoon ground allspice

- 3 tablespoon canola oil

- 2 tablespoons 1% low fat milk

- 1 large egg

- Cooking spray

Method

1. Preheat the oven to 400 degrees. Pour flour into dry measuring cups and then level them with a knife. Now take flour and add to it dark brown sugar, baking powder, teaspoon salt, ground cinnamon and ground allspice. Take a small bowl and add zucchini. To this, add canola oil, low fat milk, melted butter, vanilla milk and egg.

2. Now add the zucchini mixture to the flour mixture and stir the batter thoroughly. Divide the batter evenly among 24 muffin cups and coat it with a cooking spray. Bake the dish at 400 degrees for 10 minutes.

Tips

The taste of zucchini comes best when you make sure that the batter is evenly mixed. Do not leave any clogs in between. Also, make sure that you pour the batter in an even manner inside the muffin cups.

26. Sunflower Granola Breakfast Parfaits

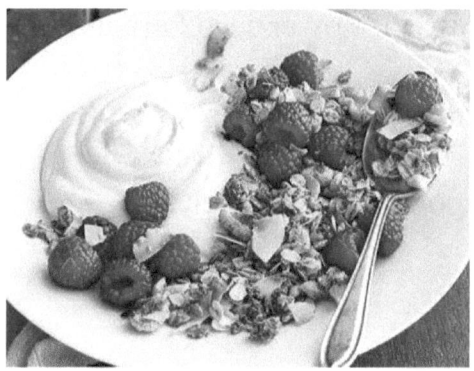

When you are looking for a great breakfast recipe, this one is definitely a good choice.

Ingredients

- 1 cup of rolled oats
- ¼ cup shredded sweetened coconut
- ½ teaspoon ground cinnamon
- 2 cups raspberries
- ¼ cup chopped walnuts
- ½ teaspoon vanilla extract
- ¼ teaspoon salt
- 2 tablespoons honey

- 4 cups plain Greek yogurt which is fat free

- ¼ cup raw sunflower seed kernels

- ¼ cup flaxseed meal

- 2 tablespoon melted butter

Method

1. Place the oven rack on the middle shelf and the boiler should be about 10 inches below it. Preheat the broiler to high. Take a baking sheet and put oats, sunflower seed kernels, sweetened coconuts, chopped walnuts, flaxseed meal, ground cinnamon and salt to it.

2. Broil the whole mixture for 3 minutes and make sure to stir it every 1 minute. Take a small bowl and combine honey, butter and vanilla. Pour the butter mixture over the oat mixture.

3. Broil granola for an additional 2 minutes. Remove granola from the oven and then let it cool in pan for another 8 minutes. Take ½ cup of yogurt and pour it into each of these 8 bowls. Top it with 1/4 cup of berries and 1/3 cup of granola

Tips

An important tip to be considered when making this dish is to ensure that you keep on stirring the mixture from time to

time. Lack of right stirring can cause the dish to be improperly cooked.

27. Swedish Meatballs

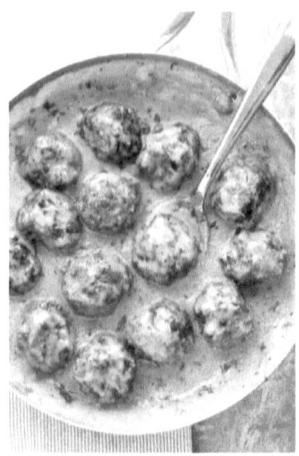

Preparing the dish takes close to 6 hours; however, we are still listing it here because you can leave it to cook for 6 hours and you can carry on with your tasks as it doesn't need a constant supervision.

Ingredients

- 1 can of beef broth
- 2 ½ lbs. of frozen meatballs
- ½ c of water
- 1 can cream of mushroom soup
- An envelope of brown gray mix
- 1 golden mushroom soup

Method

1. Take all the ingredients except the meatballs and whisk them together. Take a Crockpot and put meatballs in it.

2. Now, pour the whole mixture over the meatballs. Let it cook on low for about 6 hours.

Tips

This is one of the easiest dishes to prepare, but you need to sure that you are picking the quality of meats. Choosing inferior quality of meatballs will make a very poor dish.

28. Apple and Bacon Pita Pizzas

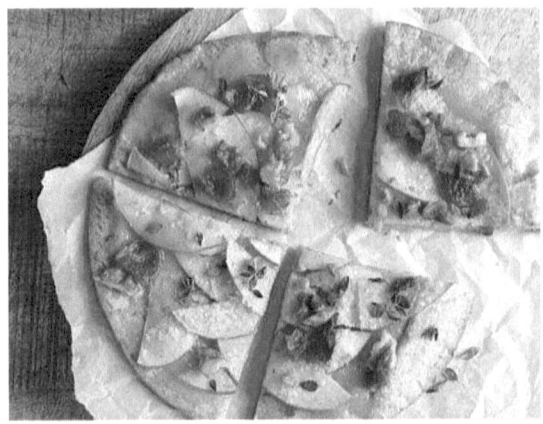

If you want to spice up your pizza by adding the right delicacy to them, this is the recipe you should not miss out on. The eclectic combination of bacon with pizza gives it a rich flavor.

Ingredients

- 4 whole wheat pitas measuring 6 inches each

- 2 cups of thinly sliced Fuji apple

- ½ cup shredded cheddar cheese

- 2 bacon slices which are apple wood smoked and are chopped and cooked thoroughly

- Tablespoons of grated parmesan cheese, fresh

- 2 teaspoons olive oil

- 1 teaspoon of fresh thyme, evenly chopped

- 2 tablespoons of walnut that are chopped and toasted

Method

1. Preheat the broiler high. Take pitas and broil them for a minute until they turn little golden in color. Now remove them from the oven and flip them very carefully. Sprinkle a little olive oil, taking care that you do it evenly.

2. Also, make it a point to sprinkle cheddar over the pitas. Take apple slices and arrange them nicely over cheese. Now, sprinkle parmesan cheese thyme, bacon and walnuts over the apples. Return to the oven and broil it for a couple of minutes.

Tips

This is one of the tastiest flavors of pizza for those who love bacon. You should be careful when you are sprinkling the ingredients because tossing them unevenly can hamper the overall taste of the pizza.

29. Peach and Blueberry Oatmeal

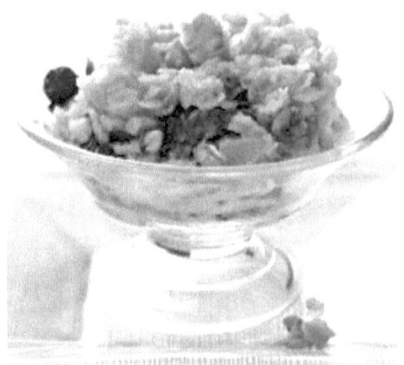

Oatmeal is one of the best dishes you could possibly have. When you choose peach and blueberry oatmeal, the way the two flavors blend into each other is delicious.

Ingredients

- 3 cups steel cut oats
- 1 pound of unsweetened fresh peaches
- 8 cups water
- 2 cups frozen blueberries
- 1 ½ teaspoon sea salt
- 1 tablespoon real vanilla
- 2 teaspoons ground cinnamon

Method

1. Spray the slow cooker with cooking spray. Take a Crockpot and combine all other remaining ingredients in it.

2. When you combine everything, it is likely that the cinnamon and fruit is probably going to rise to the top. It is alright and not a reason to worry. Let it cook on low for 8 hours. Take a sweetener of your choice which could be butter or milk and serve it along with it.

Tips

If you are skeptical of the total calorie count which you are consuming, we would request you to take gluten free oats and vanilla. Also, you can pick dairy free milk as well as it helps in cutting your calorie count.

30. Baked Apples

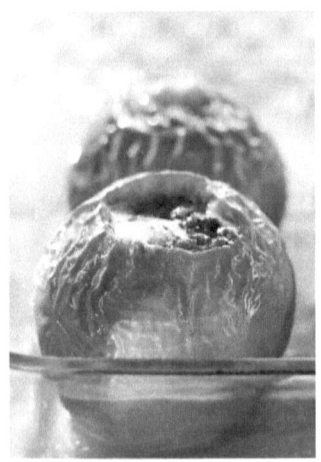

It is no surprise that apple is one of the most nutrient rich food. However, this doesn't make it a great favorite among children. This recipe for baked apple will make apples a lot tastier.

Ingredients

- 5 peeled, sliced apples
- 2 tablespoon cornstarch
- ¼ cup brown sugar
- 1 tablespoon cubed butter
- 1/8 tablespoon ground nutmeg
- ¼ cup brown sugar

- ½ cup apple juice

- ¼ cup granulated sugar

- ½ teaspoon vanilla

Method

1. Take the peeled apple and slice them. Take a Crockpot and add sugar, apple juice, cornstarch, cinnamon, vanilla, apple, nutmeg and stir them thoroughly.

2. Take butter and place it over the apples. Cook the whole mixture on high for nearly 1 ½ hours. Make sure to stir the mixture while cooking.

Tips

Make it a point to use the best apples. Fuji apples are an excellent choice as they are juicy and taste really good. If you have a sweet tooth, you can pick your favorite dessert and serve the baked apples with it.

31. Pumpkin Risotto

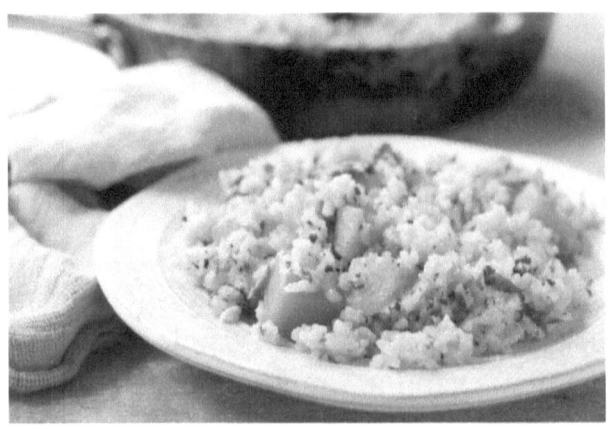

This is an excellent health dish, especially during the summers. The taste of pumpkin is delectable and when cooked in the right manner, this dish can fill your stomach completely.

Ingredients

- 1 2/3 cup Arborio rice
- 1 can pumpkin puree weighing 15 oz.
- 2 minced sage leaves
- 3 tablespoon extra-virgin olive oil
- ½ cup freshly grated parmesan cheese
- 2 small rosemary branches. Make sure that the leaves are removed and properly minced.

- 1 finely diced clove garlic

- 1 carton chicken broth weighing 32 oz.

- ½ medium sized onion which has been finely diced.

Method

1. Take a small sauté pan and then add diced onion and garlic along with 2 teaspoons of olive oil and sauté it until you spot a slightly golden color. Keep it aside now. Take the remaining olive oil and pour it in a small 3-quart Crockpot.

2. Take the sautéed onion mixture along with canned pumpkin, chicken north, Arborio rice and then stir them thoroughly. Cover the whole mixture and cook it on low for 4 hours. Stir the whole mixture after a couple of hours. When the dish has been cooked, stir it by adding the grated parmesan cheese and enjoy to the fullest.

Tips

If you want a vegetarian serving, you can always replace the chicken broth with a vegetable broth. Also, the cooking time is crucial, and you should not rush through the preparation.

32. Raspberry Ricotta Cake

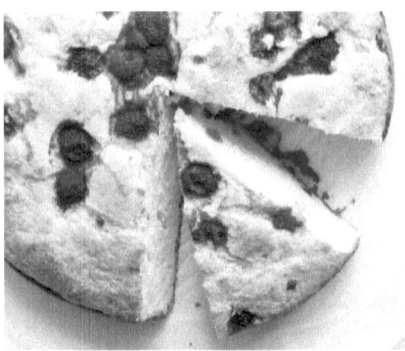

No matter how efficient a cook you are, but as long as you are unable to make a dessert, you will truly fail to impress. This is why we have one of the best cake recipes here which is going to leave everyone asking for more.

Ingredients

- 3 large eggs

- ½ teaspoon vanilla extract

- Nonstick vegetable oil spray

- 1 ½ cups ricotta

- 1 cup sugar

- ¾ teaspoon kosher salt

- ½ cup melted unsalted butter

- 2 teaspoons baking powder

- 1 ½ cups all-purpose flour

- 1 cup frozen raspberries

Method

1. Preheat the oven to 350 degrees. Take a cake pan having 9 inches diameter. Line it with a parchment paper and coat it with nonstick spray. Take a large bowl and mix flour, baking powder, sugar powder and salt. Take a medium bowl and mix eggs, vanilla and ricotta making it a smooth paste. Fold in all the dry ingredients in it.

2. Now fold in butter to the whole mixture. Add ¾ cup raspberries and make sure that you do not crush the berries when you are folding it to the mix. Take the pan and scrape butter into it. Pour the leftover raspberries over the top. Bake the whole fish until it assumes a golden-brown color. It should approximately take 50 to 60 minutes. Let it cool for 20 minutes. The cake is ready to be served.

Tips

You have to be gentle with the way you handle the raspberries. It is easy to crush it and if it so happens, it can hamper the appeal of the dish. You can also bake the cake a couple of days before and store it at room temperature. The cake will still be fresh to eat.

33. Cashew Chicken

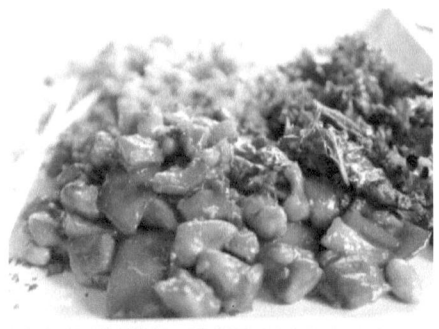

The combination of chicken and cashew is always exotic and tastes delicious. Chicken is very rich in protein and is ideal for growing children. When you are preparing this dish at home, you can curtail the sodium amount and use more frozen produce to keep the calorie count in check.

Ingredients

- 2 chicken breasts that have been cut into smaller pieces
- 1 cup of sliced carrots
- ½ cup soy sauce
- 1 tablespoon ginger paste
- ½ cup water
- ½ cup cashews. They can be ether chopped or even whole

- 3 tablespoons of ketchup
- 1 to 2 cups of broccoli, frozen
- minced garlic clove
- 4 tablespoons of rice wine vinegar
- ¼ teaspoons of red pepper flakes
- 1 tablespoon olive oil
- 1 tablespoon of brown sugar
- Salt and pepper as per requirements

Method

1. Take a Crockpot and layer the chicken along with the cashews and vegetables. Combine all other remaining ingredients except water. Make sure to pour them over chicken in your Crockpot.
2. Now add water to the mixture to make sure that it is complexly covered. Cook the whole mix for 2 to 4 hours n high.

Tips

Make sure not to hurry with the cooking time because the chicken needs to really be cooked thoroughly. Also, it is best advised to choose unsalted cashew as they seem to work best. Using salted cashews can lead to an over-salted dish.

34. Peanut Butter Hummus Along with Cucumber Dips

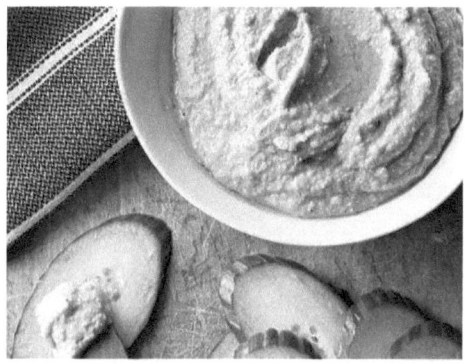

The summer season is best for those who love cucumber. This is an excellent recipe for making a quick summer dish that can help you stay full. Cucumber doesn't contribute to your calorie intake and is a healthy choice.

Ingredients

- 3 tablespoons of creamy peanut butter

- 1 cucumber which has been cut into 1/4-inch slices, 48 in number.

- ½ teaspoon ground cumin

- 7 tablespoons water

- 1 minced garlic clove

- ½ teaspoon black pepper

- 1 can chickpeas measuring 15 ½ ounces. Make sure they are rinsed and drained.
- 3 tablespoons of fresh lemon juice
- 2 teaspoons along with 1 tablespoon of olive oil
- 3/8 teaspoon kosher salt

Method

1. Take a microwave safe bowl and place peanut butter at high for 20 seconds. Now take a food processor and pour lemon juice, chickpeas, ground cumin, olive oil, kosher salt, black pepper and garlic cove and mix it together along with peanut butter.

2. When the food processor is running, make it a pint to slowly pour in water and keep on processing it until it turns smooth. Serve the dish along with cucumber.

Tips

Make it a point to process the mixture thoroughly. You have to be careful when adding water as you should not add too much water and make the whole dish very thin.

Final Words

I would like to thank you for downloading my book and I hope I have been able to help you and educate you about something new.

If you have enjoyed this book and would like to share your positive thoughts, could you please take 30 seconds of your time to go back and give me a review on my Amazon book page!

I greatly appreciate seeing these reviews because it helps me share my hard work!

Again, thank you and I wish you all the best with your cooking journey!

Last Chance to Get YOUR Bonus!

FOR A LIMITED TIME ONLY – Get Olivia's best-selling book *"The #1 Cookbook: Over 170+ of the Most Popular Recipes Across 7 Different Cuisines!"* absolutely FREE!

Readers have absolutely loved this book because of the wide variety of recipes. It is highly recommended you check these recipes out and see what you can add to your home menu!

Once again, as a big thank-you for downloading this book, I'd like to offer it to you *100% FREE for a LIMITED TIME ONLY!*

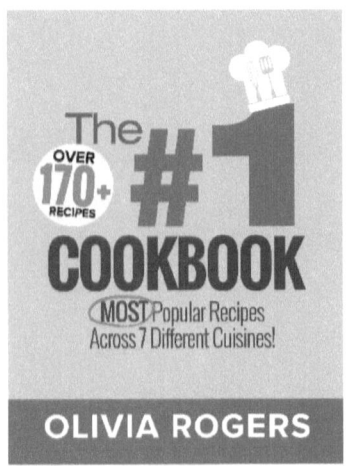

Get your free copy at:

TheMenuAtHome.com/Bonus

Disclaimer

This book and related site provides recipe and food advice in an informative and educational manner only, with information that is general in nature and that is not specific to you, the reader. The contents of this book and related site are intended to assist you and other readers in your personal efforts. Consult your physician or nutritionist regarding the applicability of any information provided in our information to you.

Nothing in this book should be construed as personal advice or diagnosis, and must not be used in this manner. The information provided about conditions is general in nature. This information does not cover all possible uses, actions, precautions, side-effects, or interactions of medicines, or medical procedures. The information in this site should not be considered as complete and does not cover all diseases, ailments, physical conditions, or their treatment.

No Warranties: The authors and publishers don't guarantee or warrant the quality, accuracy, completeness, timeliness, appropriateness or suitability of the information in this book, or of any product or services referenced by this site.

The information in this site is provided on an "as is" basis and the authors and publishers make no representations or warranties of any kind with respect to this information.

This site may contain inaccuracies, typographical errors, or other errors.

Liability Disclaimer: The publishers, authors, and other parties involved in the creation, production, provision of information, or delivery of this site specifically disclaim any responsibility, and shall not be held liable for any damages, claims, injuries, losses, liabilities, costs, or obligations including any direct, indirect, special, incidental, or consequences damages (collectively known as "Damages") whatsoever and howsoever caused, arising out of, or in connection with the use or misuse of the site and the information contained within it, whether such Damages arise in contract, tort, negligence, equity, statute law, or by way of other legal theory.

www.ingramcontent.com/pod-product-compliance
Lightning Source LLC
Chambersburg PA
CBHW021130080526
44587CB00012B/1216